Six Pack Abs in Six Easy Steps

Ab Workout

Table of Contents

Introduction

We asked women to tell us which part of man's body they find the most attractive. In most cases, the answer was stomach. Nice, flat stomach is considered beautiful also by men. Apart from looking sexy, six pack abs are also a sign that the body is healthy. The person with no belly fat is most likely to have a good blood pressure, strong hearth and no diabetes. These are all health issues that can be spotted just by looking at a person's tummy. Check out my website http://www.losingbellyfatmission.com

The belly is perhaps the hardest body region to lose fat from. Even if your body fat percentage is low, you might not have the six pack abs. They are only reserved for the most persistent ones. Or not? Maybe only a small number of people has amazing six packs, because only a few know what to do to get them. Hard workouts are not enough; there is a number of factors that influences the loss of belly fat.

It is often said that six packs are made in the kitchen, not gym. There's a lot of truth to that, but one needs a lot more than just eating healthy. Luckily for you, you've downloaded this book, in which we discuss all problems regarding belly fat. If you follow advices from this eBook, you're almost a 100 percent guaranteed to get a nice set of abs in no longer than six weeks. So the first step is to read the book and find out how to get abs. We hope you'll enjoy it!

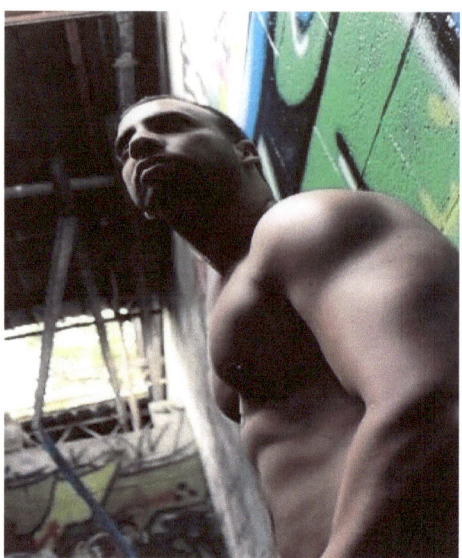

Chapter 1 – Step One: Abs Workout

Although the bigger part of the six pack abs program is diet, it's completely pointless if you do not work out regularly. There are many ways to lose the belly fat, some of which we are going to explore in this chapter. First things first – let's explain how fat burning works. The fact is that most people believe you can lose fat from a certain region only, but that's far from the truth. Forget about those "magic" gadgets for abs that apparently you just need to turn on and they'll burn the fat for you. Fat burning is all about calories. Fat is actually the energy stored by our bodies to be used when needed. So, you're either burning the fat from all regions of the body or none. It's true, though, that you're more likely to lose fat from other parts than stomach, but that's because there's usually more fat accumulated on buttocks than on your belly.

At this point, you're probably asking yourself not only how to lose belly fat, but also fat from other parts of the body. As we mentioned, fat is used as energy when body needs it. Stick to 2,000 calories diet and your body will need energy only when you're working out. With that diet regime, all energy used during a physical activity will be the one coming from body fat.

A kilogram of fat contains 9,000 calories, which means it is very hard to burn it, even with a 2,000 calories diet. Here is an example list with most popular types of fitness activities and the amount of calories they burn per hour:

- Cycling: between 350 and 500 calories
- Jogging: about 400 calories
- Jumping rope: 650 calories
- Rowing: 700 calories
- Swimming: between 550 and 800 calories
- Running up stairs: 850 calories

So, depending on the amount of fat you have in your body, you might have to do a lot of fitness in order to get six packs.

Be aware that, the more lean muscle you have, the more calories you need. That means that building lean muscle in your abdomen will result in burning more fat. Because of that, you need to do exercises designed for strong abs, together with aerobic exercises. You could separate these two exercise types into two parts. Do one early in the morning, the other in the late afternoon. In fact, the research has shown that the best part of the day for workout is after you get up and late in the afternoon, 4-5 hours before you usually go to bed.

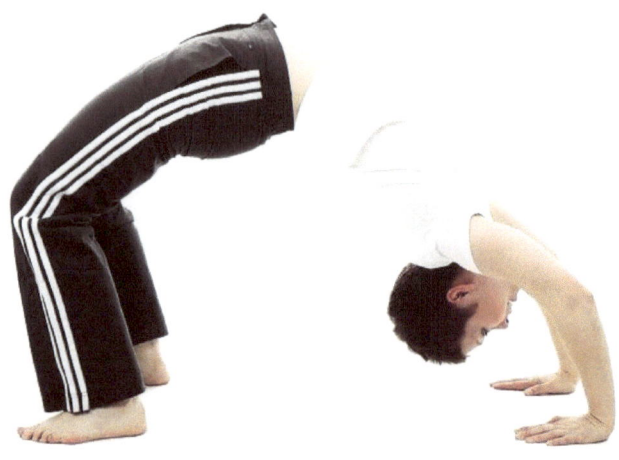

Chapter 2 – Five Best Exercises for Flat Stomach

Bicycle Crunch

Research conducted by the San Diego University has shown that this exercise puts abs to work nearly 250% more than regular crunches.

How it's done:

- Lie on your back, lift your feet off the ground and gently fold them in the knees. Keep your hands behind your head.
- While moving one knee toward your chest, simultaneously move the opposite elbow toward the knee. Alternately switch left and right knees, as well as the elbows.
- Do 2 -3 series of 10-20 repetitions.

Hanging Leg Raises

An even better exercise than bicycle crunch is the hanging leg raises. It engages every of the ab muscles, but especially the lower abs.

 How it's done:

- Hold on the shaft with your hands, so that your feet do not touch the ground

- Lift the legs up (bent at the knees), just over waist level. Exhale while you're lifting the legs up and inhale while you're putting them down.
- Do two sets of 10-15 repetitions.

Reverse Crunch

The name was coined to illustrate the movement during this exercise which involves raising the legs and lower torso, as opposed to the usual raising the upper body during the work on the abs.

How it's done:

- Get on the ground or a bench and straighten the arms along the body.
- Bring your knees to the chest so your legs would be bent at 90 degrees at the knees
- By contracting the abs, lift your hips up, straightening your legs
- Do three sets of 20 repetitions

Side Crunch

One of the most annoying areas where the fat is accumulated is the hip area. That's why you need to vigorously work on side abs and this is the best exercise for them.

How it's done:

- Lie down sideways, so that one of your shoulders and one buttock will be touching the ground. Your knees should be pressed against one another
- Put your hands behind your head and start lifting the abdomen until you create a 90 degree angle with the legs.
- Apart from simply raising your body, you need to put effort in also keeping the balance. Breathe out while lifting the body and exhale as you're getting back down
- Do 5-8 repetitions before switching sides. Try to do no less than 3 sets.

Dragon Flag

If you watched the fourth installment of the epic saga of Rocky, you surely remember those amazing exercises practiced by the American hero in preparation for a showdown with his Soviet nemesis, Ivan Drago. This exercise is one of the best lower ab workouts.

- Lie down on the ground, with your whole back pressed against the floor
- You need to have smothering to grab on to with your hands, behind your head
- Now lift the legs as high as possible and, if you can, try to lift the lower back as well

- Stay at the highest point for a moment, before slowly putting the legs back on the floor
- Do at least 5 repetitions in each series

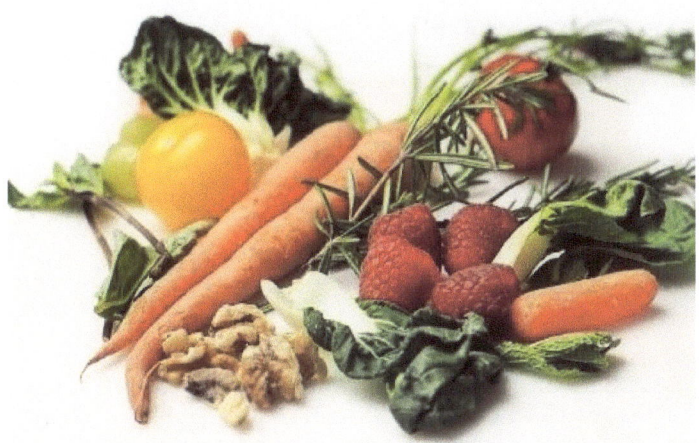

Chapter 3 - Step Two: Diet Plans

Exercising is pointless if you keep on eating unhealthy food. In fact, it can make the things even worse. The combination of sugary drinks and carb-rich fast food with hard workout will not result in losing fat and getting a hot body. It will do the opposite. You will not gain lean muscle, but pure mass. Instead of looking like a model, you'll look like a sumo wrestler. So, the thing you should do now is to decide whether you really want to get a six pack or not. If you do, you'll need to say farewell to sweets, snacks and sodas for at least a few weeks.

There are lots of diet plans you can find online, which claim to help loosing excessive fat. They differ in many things, but basically their main principle includes eating healthy protein rich food, consuming enough omega fatty acids and avoiding too much carbs.

In the next month and a half the core of your diet should be fish. When comparing the nations around the world, we found that the most healthy ones are those where fish consumption is prominent. The leanest nations in the world, traditionally eat a lot of seafood. Tuna and salmon, are both rich in protein, have almost no carbs and have a medium amount of fat, mostly comprised of omega fatty acids.

Vegetables are also your allies in fighting persistent body fat. But, not all veggies are good for dieting. Some of them have too much carbohydrates, which your body will use for energy, instead of using the stored fat. So, you will have to through away all sorts of grains, including the cereal which is claimed to be healthy and good for weight loss. You will also need to stop eating legumes and nuts, all of which are rich with carbs. Instead, include low-carb vegetables in your diet. Here is a list of vegetables you should eat on daily basis:

- Broccoli
- Cabbage
- Celery
- Mushrooms
- Spinach
- Cauliflower
- Spring onion
- Radish
- Beetroot
- Lettuce

You will not get fat by eating fatty foods, just like you won't turn green by eating lettuce. But not all types of fats and oils are the same. You need to avoid using refined and use virgin oils instead. Virgin olive and coconut oil will help you lose weight, but will also increase the amount of good cholesterol, thus protecting your heart and blood vessels.

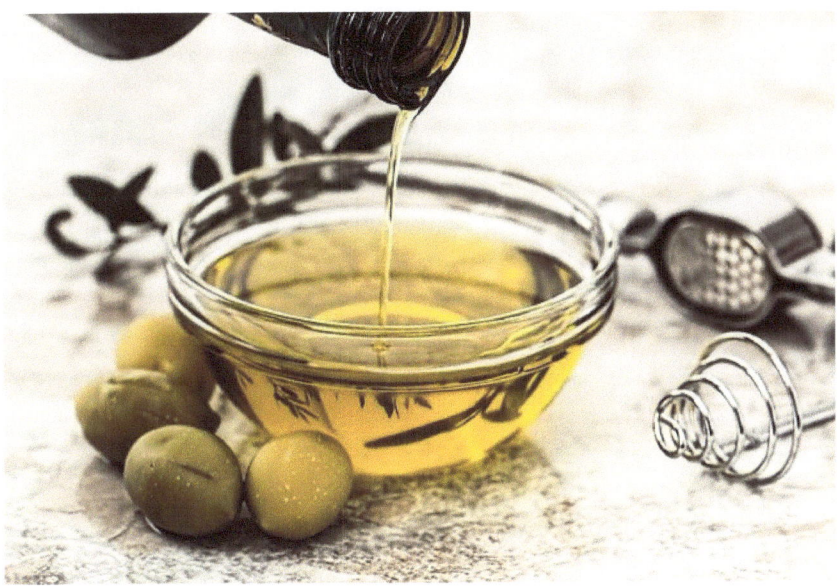

Chapter 4 – Mediterranean Diet

People living in the Mediterranean countries are known for living healthy and long. It might be the climate, but it's more likely to have to do with their diet. In fact, the main foods Mediterranean people use are seafood, poultry, olive oil and wine. Basically the same foods are used in other countries with healthy citizens, like Japan and Finland.

With water making two thirds of the planet, you might think that fish and seafood are the most popular sources of protein in human diet. Nope - people tend to eat much more pork than fish. But, that should change as fish has way better amino acid profile than pork and much higher amount of healthy fats. On top of that, fish can be really tasty. There are a lot of fish special out there in the sea, so choose from tuna, cod, halibut, haddock, etc.

Poultry farming is common in Mediterranean countries. It probably has to do with the terrain as it is much easier to breed chickens on steep mountains and small islands than cows and pigs. Speaking of Mediterranean islands, we need to take a closer look at Greece. There are lots of Greek islands in the Aegean Sea where living up to a hundred years of age is not uncommon. If you examine their diet, you will see that apart from eating fish and olive oil, they're also consuming dairy on daily basis. This country is known for Greek yogurt and Feta cheese, all of which you can use in your diet. These foods are rich in healthy fats and protein, while have a small amount of carbohydrates. On top of that, fermented milk products are claimed to help with all sorts of health issues, from kidney diseases to fat burning.

Greece, Italy, Spain and France, all claim they have the best olive oil in the world. Whichever you choose, you will not make a wrong choice. Olive oil is a super-food, helping you with all kinds of issues. It will accelerate your metabolism and help you burn the fat more quickly.

Apart from olive oil, Mediterranean countries are also known for being great in wine making. French and Italian wines are thought of as the best on the planet, while Spanish sangria is taking the world by storm. But you need to be very careful with wine and drink it moderately. Wine contains sugars, so you shouldn't drink more than a glass of it per week. That's more than enough to get all of the benefits from it, such as strengthening the heart muscle.

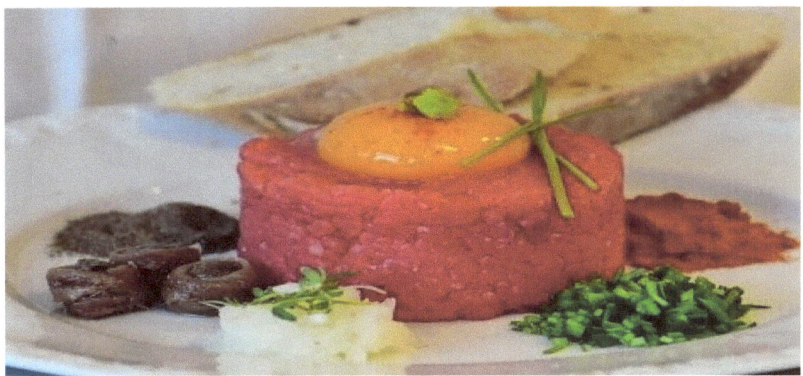

Chapter 5 – Low Carb Diet

Low Carb High Fat Diet or LCHF is based on the 65-25-10 principle, meaning that 65 percent of total calories you consume over a course of a day should come from fats, 25 percent from protein and only 10 percent from carbohydrates. At first glance, this might seem too hard to do, especially if your regular diet consists of a lot of pastries. But there are some changes in your diet to get as close to the ratio as possible.

First of all, throw away these foods from your kitchen:

- Sodas
- Alcohol beverages like bear, for example
- Sunflower oil and margarine
- Soy products
- Meat products like hotdogs and salami
- Grains and cereals
- Sweets and snacks
- Potatoes, beans, nuts and legumes
- Bananas, apples, oranges and other fruits with high amount of sugar

These are the foods you should start eating a lot more:

- Seafood
- Lean red meat
- Chicken breast
- Eggs
- Cheese
- Citrus fruits, including lemon, grapefruit, etc.
- Yogurt, kefir, sour cream
- Virgin olive and coconut oil
- Pork fat
- All kinds of spices
- Tea (green, black and white)

If you still fail to consume enough fat, you can always use supplements such as pills with omega fatty oils or fish oil made from cod liver.

Apart from LCHF diet program, there are also a lot of other diets that are based on similar principles. Those include the Atkins Diet, Dukan Diet, ITG Diet, South Beach Diet and Stillman Diet.

Chapter 6 – Step Three: Balancing Your Hormones

Sometimes the most rigorous diet regime and tentative exercises will not help you lose weight. In that case, your hormones are certainly the culprit. Failing to lose fat can be a sign of hormone imbalance. It can occur in our bodies for many reasons. Women can get it in the adolescence or after menopause, or even during pregnancy. In men, the hormone imbalance can be caused by years on unhealthy lifestyle, anabolic steroid abuse and high alcohol consumption, among many other reasons.

Whatever the reason might be, you need to tackle the problem in order to help your body function properly and eventually even lose excessive fat. In most cases, insulin is the problem. Your body does not process sugars and carbs, turning them into energy but into fat reserve. First you got to do in this case is to decrease the consumption of sugary foods. Once you fix your diet regime, the next step is to use supplements and foods that help regulating blood sugar levels and insulin.

Spices are the key. These herbs have a lot of nutrients that help your body produce enough insulin and set the hormone levels in the best ratio.   Cinnamon is perhaps the best solution for setting the insulin levels right. You can use this spice for all kinds of dishes and beverages. For example, you can put it in your coffee or tea, like people in Latin America do, or, you can add it to chicken breasts when making tikka masala and other dishes from Indian cuisine.

You can also make tea from various herbs that have good effect on balancing the levels of hormones. Marigold is great for curbing the estrogen running wild. To increase your testosterone levels, you can drink tea made from Tribulus Terrestiris, a plant native to Bulgaria. To fight stress hormone, drink tea made from St. John's Worth.

Here is a list of spices and herbs that are proven to be effective in treating hormone imbalance:

- Cinnamon
- Black pepper
- Cayenne pepper
- Parsley
- Oregano
- Dill
- Turmeric
- Coriander
- Cardamom
- Nutmeg
- Garlic
- Marigold

- Chamomile
- Bearberry
- Basil
- Menthol
- Ginger

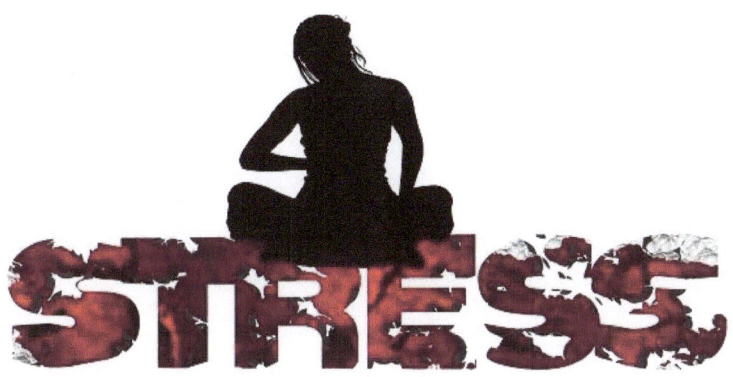

Chapter 7 – Step Four: Fighting Stress to Lose Belly Fat

You've probably heard people calling stress as the issue of the modern days. Stress in a common cause of many diseases, including those most serious ones like cancer. Fighting stress really means saving lives. So, if you have a stressful job or intense personal life, the chances are that you have fat accumulated on your belly and the hips. You can burn that fat and get six packs by working out vigorously and eating a healthy diet, but if you don't remove the thing that causes stress, the fat will keep coming back.

But, what are you supposed to do if you can locate the thing that is stressing you out, but you can't do anything to avoid it? Like having a stressful job, but needing the money. The solution is to counter it with good thing. Life is a mixture of good and bad thing, so for every stressful situation, create one happy situation. If your job is annoying, find a hobby that will make you relaxed. If the boss gets on your nerves, hang out after work with people who make you laugh.

A great way to fight stress is physical activity. Exercise increases the amount of serotonin, the hormone of happiness. So, you shouldn't think twice about enrolling in fitness program. Yoga could be even better solution for you as meditation and stretching exercises that are part of this practice are confirmed to do well for both your mind and the body.

Perhaps, your best option would be to start playing some kind of sport. That will combine all the stress-fighting factors, including exercising and hanging out with people. In fact, sport can grow from being just a healthy hobby to being one of the most important parts of your life. You'll see how the time passes fast even if you're doing the most boring work, if your mind is set on some kind of sport.

You can choose any kind of sport you wish, the sky is the limit! Still, our recommendation is to go for a team sport. If you chose a sport like boxing or tennis, you'll definitely have quite a lot of fun and will be engaged physically. But, if you decide on a team sport like hockey, football or basketball, you will also make a lot of new friends.

Sport is probably the best way to fight stress, but there are plenty more other activities that can help you feel better and subsequently improve your overall health, including losing the belly fat. Did you know that when your brain is working hard, you're burning the calories? So, nothing's stopping you enrolling in a crafts class. Learn how to draw or do clay sculptures. An even better option is to learn a new language. Scientific research has shown that people who speak more than one language are less likely to develop Alzheimer's disease when they get old.

Of course, you can also fight stress with a good diet. Apart from healthy diet regime, you need to start consuming a few other foods. Valerian root is amazing for helping you sleep better and stop being anxious. Same goes for St. John's Worth, which has the ability to calm you down. Cocoa is also proved to help secreting the happiness hormone.

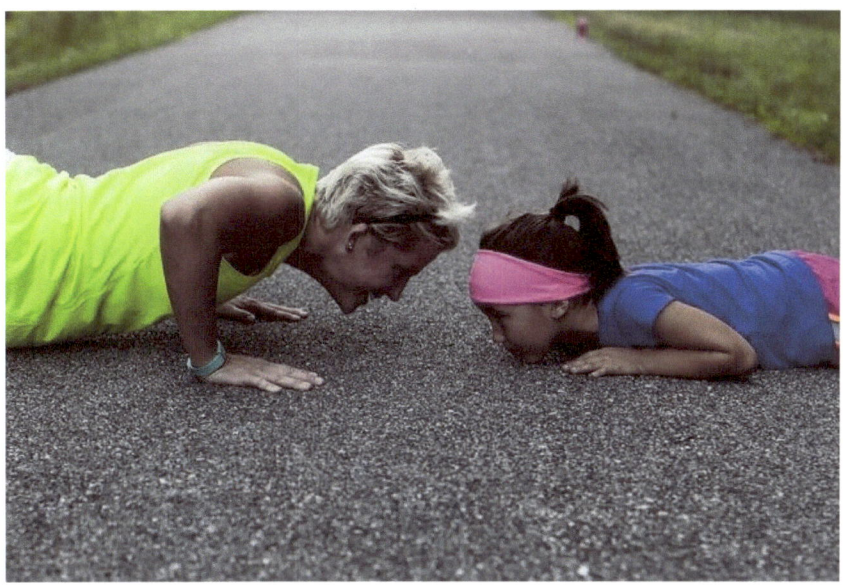

Chapter 8 – Step Five: Implementing Healthy Life Regime

At first look, you might think that changing your diet is going to be very hard and expensive process. Still, that can't be further from the truth. Instead of paying for a burger in a fast food restaurant, you can make your own meal. Not only will you choose the healthiest ingredients, you will also use only those that you like the most. Apart from the taste, the homemade meal is bound to be cheaper than the one from a fast food restaurant.

Say goodbye to sodas and every kind of carbonated drink. Sodas are full of sugar and even the light versions that are claimed to be calorie-free, are not good for you. They contain other substances, which can have potentially bad effect on your body leading to other life threatening illnesses. Instead of soft drinks, you can always choose lemonade or a tea. Tea is a great solution for you. You can drink black tea in the morning, because it has the highest amount of caffeine of all types of tea. You can drink green during the day, to keep you fresh and you can drink white tea in the evening as it has very small amount of caffeine.

Coffee is okay in small amounts, while in large amounts it can mess up your hormone balance. Avoid drinking it in the evening as the high amount of caffeine can keep awake. Avoid using the other stimulants as well, like energy drinks. Of course, forget about using illegal substances and try to lower the amount of alcohol. You can drink a couple of beers every now and then, but be aware that alcohol has no nutritional value for the body, which treats it as a poison. Once it enters our system, our liver works hard to break it to smaller molecules, so the body could throw it away.

Stress and its product, hormone named cortisol is your biggest enemy. Fight it anytime, anyplace. In the previous chapter, we explained what you can do in order to alleviate the symptoms of stress, so do your best to stick to them. Join a sport club, develop a hobby and hang out with interesting people will certainly benefit both your mind and your body.

Make exercise your daily routine. Psychologists have said many times that only three weeks are needed to develop any kind of habit. So, try your best not to skip trainings for at least first 21 days. It'll get easier with time. In fact, we're sure that when you see the results – six packs, you'll never want to stop working out.

Here are a few simple things you can do every day that can change your life for the better:

- Drink a glass of lukewarm water every morning as soon as you wake up. The water will kick-start your body, waking you up.
- Sleep in the dark. Studies have shown that the level of melatonin in a human body, a hormone that gets secreted only during night, has decreased in the last half a century. The reason for that is that people started using more and more technology. So, don't let the TV put you to sleep. Turn it off at least an hour before going to bed. Instead, read a book or a magazine or even better, listen to radio, in dark.
- Let the sunshine in as soon as you get up as the natural light will wake your body up.
- Take a hot'n'cold shower every morning. Alternately switch from hot water to cold as it will have a great effect on your blood vessels, improving the circulation and protecting you from blood pressure problems in the long term.
- Eat a big and healthy breakfast. It takes about 5 hours for food to pass through human body. So, have that in mind to set the time of your meals. Let's say you're awake 16-17 hours each day, that means that you need between three and four meals, the first ideally in the first hour after you wake up, the dinner at least three hours before going to bed.

- If you can, walk to your work instead of driving or going by bus. Not only is walking a type of physical activity, it also can spark creativity. As many people before you, you can also find solutions appear before you while walking.
- Laugh as much as you can. The whole point of life is being happy, so use every opportunity to hang out with people who make you laugh. But there's much more to laughing than just making you happy. It is a fact that laughing accelerates the metabolism.
- Read more and learn new things every day. If you don't use your brain as much as you should, you can start feeling depressed. Depression induced by boredom is a common matter, but you can easily fight it just by reading an interesting book now and then.

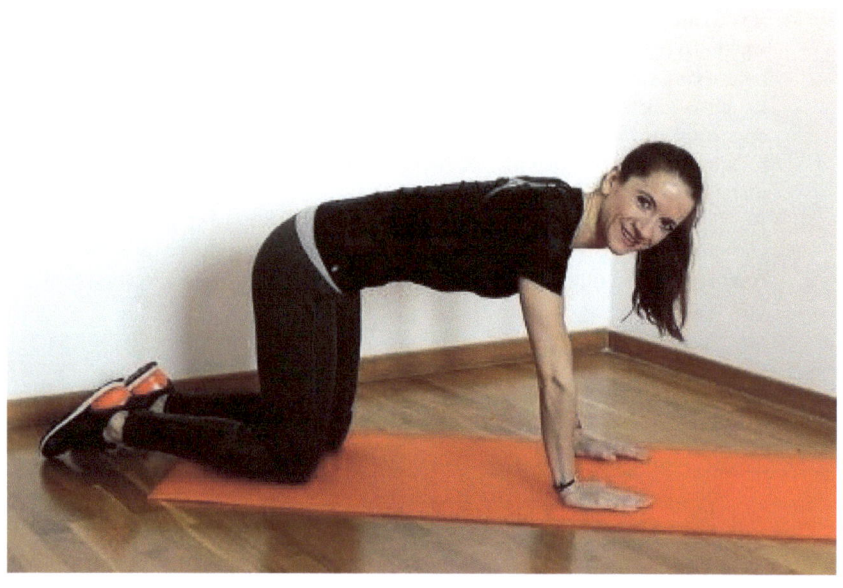

Chapter 9 – Step Six: Making Sure You Never Lose Six Packs

Same as all muscles, abs also require a lot of work. It is true that you can get six packs in only six weeks, but your work must not stop at that point. Fat goes easily, but also comes back easily. That's why you must not stop with your healthy diet regime once you get a nice set of abs. You also should not stop working out on regular basis, even after the six week program is completed, for the same reasons.

If you are thinking about the future, your long term abs plan should be a healthy diet and a good workout routine. But, if you really want to make sure, you will not lose them, you need to do the 6-week program thoroughly. The bigger the muscles, the more energy they need. That means that if you have strong core muscles, fat will not store at that region easily. So, one of your short-term plans should be to gain lean muscle mass in the abdomen. Good diet and ab exercises you can find in this book should do the job.

If you stick to the diet programs we've mentioned already in this eBook, then you have nothing to worry about. Still, if you want to be a hundred percent sure your six packs abs will last for a long period and on top of that, you are open to spending a bit of money, then you should think about buying a whey protein powder. There are a lot of them on the market, varying a lot in terms of price and quality. If you decide to buy one for you, look for a hydrolyzed whey powder as that type contains the proteins with the best kind of amino acid profile. Usually, whey protein powder contains between 80 and 90 percent of protein, so these products can be useful in supplementing your diet in order to reach the wanted protein amount.

Apart from building muscle, you also need to make sure your metabolism is fast enough to burn calories instead of storing them. You can achieve this only by leading a healthy life and eating healthy foods. On top of that, you can make it even better by eating 5-6 smaller meals each day. That will keep your body digesting food all the time, thus working the whole day. Your metabolism will also accelerate if you hydrate with enough water. Usually, only a few glasses are enough for the body to function normally, but if you wish to speed it up, double the amount.

Finally, in order to have a sexy abdomen, you can cheat a bit. The fact is that a body will appear more muscular if it's tanned, even if the tape measure says different. So, a bit of sunbathing will not do you any harm and will surely make you look and feel hotter. Try to limit your expose to no more than 20 minute to an hour a day, but not between the hours of 10am – 2pm when the sun is most intense. There can be other problems developed from too much sun exposure, mainly skin cancer.

Conclusion

Here are some of the most important take away from this book. Remember, practice makes perfect with anything in time.

Getting six pack abs has much more importance than just looking good. The abdomen shows how healthy you are, so it is out of great importance to lose the belly fat. It is proven that people with narrow waist and six packs are less prone to diseases like diabetes and all kinds of coronary issues. But, let's face it – for most of people who are looking to get six packs, the appearance is the key factor.

Whatever the reason might be, losing belly fat can have a lot of benefits, both for your mind and your body. Once you get a six pack abdomen, you'll start feeling better about yourself. That will certainly make you want to keep on doing whatever helped you get them, in this case a healthy lifestyle and regular exercise. Apart from obvious benefits, there are lots of other good things this six weeks program can do for you. Eating a healthy diet with low carbohydrates and a high enough amount of healthy fat will make improve your overall health. Your sugar level will become normal if you had problems with it prior. Same goes for the blood pressure. This type of diet will accelerate your metabolism, making you more energized and helping you sleep better.

You can get so much just by doing these relatively simple things. We encourage you to follow the diet and workout regime for six weeks and if you're satisfied with the result, keep on doing it. If not, you didn't lose anything as this program is completely safe. The ab workouts we mentioned are done by using nothing but your own weight, which eliminates any risk of injuries. Still, it is advisable to consult your personal physician before starting with the six week abs program.

Be sure that no matter how difficult this program might seem to you at this point, the hardest thing about it is the beginning. The first step is the hardest to make. You might not realize it, but you have already made it – downloading this eBook shows that you are willing to take your life in your own hands and make changes to feel and look better. From now on, everything will get easier, once you have made up your mind. The goal is there, you just need to achieve it!

Check my website http://www.losingbellyfatmission.com for regular weight loss and diet tips. I also have a series of other workout and nutritional books on Amazon.com, createspace.com and elsewhere online.

www.ingramcontent.com/pod-product-compliance
Lightning Source LLC
Chambersburg PA
CBHW050932290526
45792CB00002B/990